Worried Sick?
The Workbook

A Day by Day and Week by Week Program
For the Treatment of Health Anxiety,
For People Who Worry Too Much about their Health

By Fredric Neuman, M.D.

Simon & Brown
www.simonandbrown.com

Copyright © 2008, 2009 Fredric Neuman

ISBN-13: 978-0-9814843-5-8
ISBN-10: 0-9814843-5-2

Library of Congress Control Number: 2008928148
Library of Congress subject headings:
Health – Psychological
Compulsive Behavior
Health – Miscellanea

1.2

Author Online! To contact Dr. Neuman, please write to
info@simonandbrown.com

WORRIED SICK? THE WORKBOOK
THE TABLE OF CONTENTS

INTRODUCTION:
  The Methods of Cognitive-Behavioral Therapy
  Finding and Evaluating Patients to Form a Group

The health anxiety program at the White Plains Hospital
  The structure of the clinic
  The role of family members
  The role of the aide
    1.Discovering the nightmare fantasies of the health worrier
    2.Helping the health worrier confront frightening situations
    3.Discouraging the search for reassurance
    4.Encouraging the health worrier to live in a healthy way
    5.Helping to organize record keeping

Record Keeping
    1.Tracking physical symptoms
    2.The list of reassuring facts
    3.The list of nightmare fantasies

Clinic Meetings
  The First Clinic Meeting
    1.Definitions of hypochondriasis, somatization disorder and other
      related conditions
    2.An explanation of the causes of health anxiety
    3.The worry wheel
    4.An explanation of the six principles of treatment
    5.Problems that appear in the first week of treatment

  The Second Clinic Meeting
    Do's and Don'ts
    A typical problem of the second week of treatment
  The Third Clinic Meeting
    Typical problems of the remaining weeks of the program
  The Fourth Clinic Meeting
    Drugs vs. Herbs
  The Fifth Clinic Meeting: Diet and exercise and living in a healthy
    manner
  The Results of Treatment

Day by Day and Week by Week - A program for the treatment of Health Anxiety

In part because of reports in the media of new and threatening diseases, and, also, new forms of treatment, there are a great many people who are preoccupied by matters of health. Health worriers— people who worry too much about their health—make up a large proportion of the medical practice of most physicians. They over-utilize medical services, particularly diagnostic procedures, and, nevertheless, remain anxious, even when they are perfectly well. It is very difficult to reassure them. They may be diagnosed with obsessive-compulsive disorder or depression, or a number of other illnesses, but their condition is really better defined by the mistaken ideas they have about how and why people get sick. Similarly, they have Bad Ideas about drugs, doctors, and other related matters. Worried Sick? was written in order to describe health anxiety clearly and lay out a tested program for treatment. Bad Ideas are incorrect, but self-confirming, prejudices which lead people to behave in ways that worsen their fears. Treatment is directed to changing these behaviors so that health worriers can see the world and themselves more accurately. This kind of treatment is called cognitive-behavioral. The underlying principle is confrontation. It is necessary to confront one's fears in order to overcome them. This is not easy to do.

Worried Sick? recommends a number of explicit Do's and Don'ts, but even these are hard to follow. This workbook is intended to be a day by day and week by week guide to treatment. The program described was developed by the White Plains Hospital Anxiety and Phobia Center. One audience for this book are those professionals and paraprofessionals who wish to begin their own treatment program for health anxiety. The second, larger audience is made up of health worriers, themselves. The workbook includes forms for record-keeping, a very important part of the program, and suggestions for family members and others prepared to help. More important, it provides a step-by-step way of implementing the cognitive-behavioral exercises described in <u>Worried Sick?</u>

It is easy to set down in a few sentences the principles underlying the treatment of health anxiety, but implementing these principles in a practical program of treatment is not simple. Sometimes, as in any treatment program, one sets out to do one thing and ends up doing other things — sometimes unawares. Years ago, psychiatric residents were taught that the purpose of all psychotherapy was simply to make the unconscious conscious. It took years of training to discover what this formula meant and then how to use it in actual therapy. And then it turned out to be wrong. There are many different schools of psychotherapy. They have different theoretical rationales that grow out of different theories about the etiology of emotional and mental disorders; but in practice, viewed from the other side of a one-way mirror, or through the prism of supervision, they all end up doing the same thing. They take issue systematically with certain incorrect assumptions patients have about themselves or about the world in general. The settings may be different, even the methods may be different, but the purpose remains the same. For example, a woman may come to therapy because she is embittered and unhappy. She feels everyone treats her disrespectfully just because she is a woman. Consequently, she fights with everyone. Surely, it is true that someone may look down on her for being a woman; but surely not most people. The psychoanalyst listening to her may express doubt by raising an eyebrow or asking a question. The cognitive therapist may ask the patient to think of other possible explanations of behavior she usually interprets as showing contempt for her and, as an exercise, to write them down. The purpose of both is to get the patient to see things more realistically. The success of either treatment may depend on the relationship between the patient and the therapist, an imponderable. Similarly, there are different programs that can be designed reasonably to attack health anxiety, which is a specific set of misconceptions and prejudices. The following is one such program, modified over the years in response to problems and deficiencies that became apparent only over time.

Finding Patients to Form a Group

Patients do not readily identify themselves as hypochondriacs. Phobic persons may readily enlist in programs designed to help them. Health worriers do not. The stigma, they think, is too great. Physicians in general practice do not think to refer such patients to psychotherapists, not because they are so few and unusual, but because they are so many. With varying degrees of severity health worriers comprise a significant portion of every medical practice. If these were subtracted, some doctors joke, they would have no practice at all. They tend to handle such patients by warning them against reading about their feared illness and by performing unnecessary medical tests in hope of reassuring them. Neither strategy works. Undoubtedly, they would refer such patients for psychotherapy if they understood that there are special treatment methods that work. Unfortunately, health anxiety is viewed usually as simply a stubborn facet of personality. If it is diagnosed at all, it is usually considered and treated as depression or obsessive-compulsive disorder or as some other related condition. It is only those patients who are extremely affected by this problem, the tip of the iceberg, so to speak, who are referred to a psychiatrist for treatment. So, finding patients for a health anxiety treatment program means, first of all, reaching out to community physicians.

Other patients are self-referred. They may very well think that today's worry is justified by their current physical problems and yet still understand that in general they worry too much about their health. One might expect that the managed care system might be anxious to send additional such patients for treatment since these people are plainly in distress and since the expense of over-utilization of medical services and testing they engender would then be minimized; but that has not proven to be the case. Apparently, any new treatment idea, however inexpensive, is outside their purview.

Evaluating patients

Anyone who identifies himself or herself as worrying too much about illness is a suitable patient. It is important to discover whether a health worrier is also depressed or has an obsessive-compulsive disorder since these conditions need to be treated with antidepressant drugs. A depressed person may or may not feel sad, but will usually feel agitated and panicky or, conversely, very lethargic and withdrawn. Key elements of the syndrome are the so-called vegetative signs: a tendency toward interrupted sleep, frequent early morning awakening marked by jumpy or depressed feelings and irrational worries, a loss of appetite to the point of losing weight, or less commonly, gaining weight, a loss of interest in sex and a tendency to feel less bad as the day wears on. People so affected should be treated with drugs. Persons with obsessive-compulsive disorder have a variety of symptoms including repetitive checking, often to see if the front door is locked or if the stove is turned off, stereotyped rituals, such as hand washing or counting steps, an exaggerated concern over orderliness and symmetry, and an unease about contamination. They may be troubled by intrusive unpleasant thoughts — other than simply health worries. These patients also tend to respond to the same drugs, although less reliably. When these related conditions improve, usually in a matter of a number of weeks, patients can participate in a cognitive-behavioral treatment program for health anxiety. Most people who are willing to consider such a program for themselves turn out to belong in the program. Unfortunately, many people who belong in such a program do not come to it even though they are constantly worried about their health. They think they are truly ill or about to become ill and so they think it is natural and appropriate to worry all the time.

4

The health anxiety program at the White Plains Hospital

The clinical supervisor at the White Plains Hospital Clinic makes an initial evaluation of all patients. She takes a history which includes a determination of previous medical illnesses, use of medication, and previous psychotherapy. Often patients come to therapy already having been placed on tranquilizers without much relief of their anxiety. Some patients are already taking antidepressant drugs. Some have or have had a relatively serious disease. Often, patients have experienced unusual conditions. Some have never been sick at all. A surprising number have been told by doctors that they have a fatal illness — in error! Then, still preliminary to the first group meeting, they are asked to fill out forms A & B. For purposes of this manuscript, all forms and figures are at the end of this chapter. Typically, patients report that they are considerably affected by health anxiety. Those most troubled report that much of life is spoiled. Most check off over *50%* of the items on the Health Anxiety Scale; and some check off almost all. We try to keep the referring doctor informed about the patient's progress, but do not require medical clearance to accept a patient into the program. Nothing done in the clinic is likely to worsen any medical condition the patient may have.

The structure of the clinic

The clinic is a series of six weekly meetings, one and a half hours in length. A group of patients meet with trained aides and a group leader who is usually a psychiatrist. Cognitive-behavioral interventions, of which this program is one sort, are usually supervised by clinical psychologists; but, when making pronouncements about medical matters, someone with a medical degree is more credible. In the event such a program is run by a psychologist, physicians must be available on occasion to make the sort of medical distinctions drawn in the chapters of Worried Sick? Patients should focus on the treatment of their psychological problems; but their natural tendency is to become preoccupied instead with today's medical problems. The trained aides, or in lieu of aides, family members, help to keep the patient focused on the psychological treatment of this psychological disorder.

The Role of Family Members (see Worried Sick? Chapter 13)

Health anxiety is disturbing not only to the health worrier, but often to all the members of his or her family. Often they are dragged into a stereotyped and repetitive interchange in which they are required to answer the same questions over and over again. "Do I look pale? (or paler?)." "Does this mole look weird? (or weirder?)" "Does this look red to you? (or redder?)" "Do you think I'm running a fever?" Although couched in the form of requesting medical information (from people who are not medically informed), these questions are really designed to seek reassurance. Like any other kind of compulsive checking, they comfort only momentarily at the price of focusing the health worrier's attention further on the possibility of a medical calamity. These nagging questions reduce family members finally to halfhearted, distracted replies that do not serve to reassure even temporarily. These questions should be resisted sympathetically but firmly. Health worriers should be reminded that obsessional checking aggravates their condition. It is better for the family relationship to frustrate the health worrier in this way than to end up angry and exasperated. Ridicule, however good-natured, is not helpful. Every once in a while a health worrier is so persuasive, or family members are so suggestible, that they start to worry also. They are more likely to calm down, though, once they talk to the patient's doctor. It is a good idea for them to accompany the patient to the doctor's office for this reason and because patients, unaccompanied, are often too agitated to understand or remember exactly what the doctor said.

Another family problem attendant upon health anxiety is the tendency for these concerns to pass on to the next generation. Ideas are contagious. All of the Bad Ideas described in Worried Sick? can be conveyed in subtle ways or, sometimes, directly. It is hard for parents who worry excessively about their own health not to worry too about their children's health. It is still harder to worry without the children knowing. Constant admonitions to stay away from people who are sick exaggerate the danger of being sick. Talking about the importance of eating properly or getting a good night's sleep suggests the precariousness of good health. Some parents warn very explicitly about germs as if human beings had not evolved effective ways of warding off infection.[1] When judging which precautions are reasonable, one should be guided by the advice of a pediatrician rather than what seems to be obvious as a matter of "common sense." It is very hard for someone who is naturally fearful to avoid becoming overprotective. Family members can help.

It is possible, although difficult, for family members to help with the process of treatment. It is hard to be firm and dispassionate when someone you love is feeling bad. Guidelines for an aide or for someone acting as an aide follow.

The Role of the Aide

Before someone can be helpful in specific ways, it is important to know certain general rules. An aide must be willing to listen respectfully. Each of us has certain irrational fears that seem at first glance to be ridiculous to other people. However outlandish the ideas of a health worrier may seem, they follow logically from that person's experience. They may be wrong; but they must be understood in detail. It must become clear to the health worrier that his or her concerns are truly appreciated. It does no good, even at that point, to tell someone "You're wrong. The doctor says you're wrong. Stop worrying." Someone who feels bad should not be embarrassed or in other ways made to feel worse.

---

[1] It turns out that children who have had less than their share of minor infectious illnesses growing up are more likely to develop immunological problems later on such as autoimmune diseases.

It is possible to be encouraging and comforting without engaging in the ritual reassurances that the health worrier seeks. Someone who is not a doctor should not argue for or against a particular illness or express an opinion about the appropriateness or lack of appropriateness of a particular medication. In the guise of educating the patient, aides should not express their own theories of disease, whether they are nutritional, psychological or religious. However, since health anxiety rests in part upon a lack of proper medical information, any authoritative medical article or account relevant to the patients concerns should be brought to his or her attention <u>whether or not that account seems likely to make the patient worry more or worry less</u>. In the long run, learning more leads to worrying less.

Anyone afraid of anything is best able to confront that fear a little at a time and usually with another person there to help. But the helper must allow the fearful person to set the pace. If an aide is going to help someone afraid of visiting a hospital, it may be necessary for the two of them to spend considerable time in the lobby before walking through the hospital corridors. Just how much time depends on the patient. Health worriers are often so anxious at first they are unable to read about certain illnesses or confront particular nightmare fantasies. Even the various checking behaviors they have become enmeshed in cannot be abruptly set aside. It is important that they do these things, but not necessarily today and all at once. Aides can help them do more than they would on their own. Family members and aides can provide critical help encouraging and in other ways helping to motivate health worriers to confront all those issues that they need to in order to get well; but encouragement should not degenerate into simple nagging.

Facilitating Treatment

The following is an outline of those ways in which an aide can help in the treatment process:

Discovering the specific nightmare fantasies of the health worrier. Usually, there is a hierarchy of mental images, each scary in its own way. The fear of death or dying is unlikely to be foremost. More typically, health worriers are haunted by the thought of noticing something new on their bodies, a lump or a heart irregularity or some other sign of a potentially deadly disease. The next nightmare fantasy may be a scene in the doctor's office where the doctor is announcing the bad news. Or they might picture to themselves those moments on the telephone when they wait to hear the results of a laboratory test. As each fantasy dwindles with treatment, others become apparent. It is not always easy to find out just what health worriers are worrying about. They may talk about dying when they are really afraid of pain. They may talk about having a heart attack but really imagine themselves being raped while lying unconscious on the floor or, more often, imagine their children wandering away or being kidnapped. As described in Worried Sick?, the fear of dying may cover more primitive fears of being helpless or alone. Nightmare fantasies can be discovered by talking to the health worrier, sometimes only at length.

Encouraging strategies for dealing with the nightmare fantasies. Patients need, first of all, to be reminded just how unlikely is the particular catastrophe they are imagining. The chances of developing a particular disease at a particular age can usually be determined by looking through actuarial tables or by researching an appropriate web site on the internet. Sometimes patients have to make 500 or 10,000 marks on a large piece of paper to truly understand what one in 500 or one in 10,000 means. The habit of considering the odds should become ingrained. It is surely terrible for a young mother to suffer a heart attack, but it is comforting to know just how rare that is.

Aides and family members can help to find the one hour a day the health worrier is supposed to spend concentrating on nightmare fantasies. They can listen to an account of them or review them with the patient once they have been put down on paper. Making them explicit makes them less frightening. They can remind the health worrier of the "well, then..." that follows the "what if..." Sometimes the aide can supply other more reasonable explanations of the patient's symptoms. These will be less awful and more likely than those that preoccupy the patient.

Health worriers should try to put off worrying until that special time when they are supposed to concentrate on their fears. Aides can help teach them how to distract themselves at other times. Relaxation exercises may help but engaging in activities that command attention work better. These may include doing puzzles or even ordinary conversation. These tools work better with practice. Turning one's attention elsewhere seems impossible at first but becomes habitual after a while.

<u>Discovering and helping the health worrier confront any concrete situations they may be avoiding</u>. Among those most often encountered are the doctor's office, the examining table, particularly that of the gynecologist, syringes, the CAT scan tunnel, the hospital emergency room and hospitals in general, particularly those that care for dying patients. The aide can accompany the health worrier into these situations, starting first with those least threatening and staying long enough in that situation for the patient to calm down. The sense of mastery someone obtains by overcoming such irrational fears often spills over into other areas, making that person feel less vulnerable in general.

<u>Discouraging the search for reassurance</u>. Health worriers are allowed to check their bodies or bodily function <u>only to the extent that they are instructed to do so by their physician</u>. In almost all cases it is undesirable to take one's pulse, or examine one's sputum or nasal discharge, or urine, or stool or menstrual flow. No meaningful information is obtained in this way. The progress of skin lesions, if there are any, should be monitored by a patient only when told to do so by the doctor and certainly not every few hours. Breast

self-examination should be performed only once or twice a month. All of this is easy to say but very hard to do. The habit of feeling oneself constantly and prodding oneself is very hard to break. Aides and family members in particular can be very helpful in this regard, if only because health worriers often engage in these practices without realizing that they are doing so. Similarly, health worriers should be discouraged from asking doctors questions urgently that they know are not truly urgent. They should not ask rhetorical questions such as "are you sure?" or the same question over and over.

Health worriers do not recognize that focusing on their bodies not only worsens their preoccupations with disease but sometimes produces symptoms in and of itself. Pain can be produced by looking for it. Holding a hand very steady will cause trembling. Anyone's pulse will be accelerated by taking it. Someone trying to breath normally breathes too fast. The effect of mind on body can be demonstrated with a few exercises. If the patient is instructed to sign a piece of paper very slowly and carefully, the signature will not look like it usually does. Someone trying to walk carefully will not walk naturally. If someone looks about the room while walking slowly, a light-headed feeling is likely to be experienced. Everyone knows that itching and yawning are contagious. In such ways it may be possible to convince a health worrier that headaches, or gastric distress, or dizziness can be induced to a considerable extent just by looking for them.

Encouraging the health worrier to live in a healthy way. It is often the case that health worriers engage in unhealthy practices such as smoking or overeating or living sedentary lives despite their professed concern about their health. Sometimes, at the point of their coming to treatment for their anxiety, they can be influenced to give up these behaviors. At least they should be encouraged to exercise. With time, exercise has a noticeable effect on physical fitness which not only minimizes the risk from certain serious illnesses such as cardiovascular disease, but which also is the only direct way of altering the health worrier's underlying view of his or her health. Jogging past others of the same age makes it harder to entertain the idea that one is harboring a serious illness. Also, one is less likely to interpret a fast heartbeat and shortness of breath as a sign of illness if they are a familiar consequence of a healthy activity. Someone worried about his or her health would generally do better exercising rather than resting up.

<u>Helping to organize and review the health worrier's record keeping</u>

<u>Record Keeping</u>

Essential to any cognitive-behavioral treatment program are homework assignments and record keeping. Reading about and imagining feared diseases is distinctly unpleasant, and refraining from the persistent wish to check is also very uncomfortable. Homework is only tedious in the way homework always is. But record keeping is especially important.

One reason that health worriers maintain the fiction that certain diseases are more common than they really are is their tendency to remember every instance of the disease and forget all the times that illness seemed to threaten and turned out to be something else. Similarly, they experience a symptom and worry that it is evidence of some medical calamity, forgetting all the other times they had the same symptom without any consequence at all. They remember those facts that fit with their preconceptions and forget those that do not. Keeping records is the only way of bringing these false alarms back into memory.

One such record is the following notation which should be kept in a notebook:

12

The symptom I have:	The worry I have in Connection with this symptom:	What happened to this symptom:
For example: 1. My hand began to tremble today 2. I had a sharp pain over my forehead 4-5 times today	I think I might have multiple sclerosis. I think about the possibility of a brain tumor.	The shaking went away later that day. The pain went away after I took aspirin.

Health worriers start off by making entries into this chart a number of times each day. Subsequently, when their worries begin to trouble them less, they will make these notes less frequently. This record should be kept indefinitely. Often a patient worries about suspicious abdominal pains only to discover that in the past year just the same pain occurred a number of times and disappeared by the following day. When it has become apparent that the last 70 or 80 times a frightening symptom was marked down, nothing happened, even people who think they have been singled out by fate to get sick begin to think that most of the time even they do not get sick. Record keeping is one more exercise designed to make health worriers truly understand on a gut level what they claim to know on an intellectual level: that certain illnesses are very unlikely.

Compulsive checking makes health worriers worry more, in part because no matter how carefully one checks, there is always a nagging residual ambiguity. "That bump isn't bigger - or is it just a little bit bigger?" "That mole isn't a little darker - or is it?" "Is that tender part just a little bit more tender?" Even checking something by asking a doctor is likely to leave behind some uncertainty. But the urge to check is hard to suppress. For that reason, as an interim measure, the health worrier should compile a list of reassuring and unambiguous facts about his or her condition. Instead of feeling the tender lymph node one more time, or seeing if taking a deep breath still leads to coughing, or taking one's pulse for the umpteenth time, the health worrier can take out and review the list of reassuring facts. Here are examples of typical lists.

For a woman who worries about breast cancer:
1. I was examined last month and six months before that by my gynecologist; and she did not see any evidence of a breast cancer.
2. When I examine my own breast, I don't feel anything like a hard marble or a hard lump attached to the surrounding skin.
3. A lot of lumps, even hard lumps, in the breast are not due to cancer.
4. The chance of my developing cancer at my age is one in 580 over the next year.
5. If I do develop cancer, the chance of my being cured is 95%.
6. There are new drugs being investigated that may go a long way to preventing breast cancer.

A man who is afraid of developing a fatal cardiac arrhythmia might have this list of reassuring facts:
1. Two cardiologists have assured me that the irregular heart beat I have is not serious.
2. I have had two Holter monitor tests and neither showed any abnormal beats.
3. A normal heart can beat quickly for long periods of time without suffering injury.
4. I have not ever fainted or had any serious symptoms because of my heart irregularity.
5. The extra heart beats I have are not supposed to progress to coronary artery disease or to heart attacks.
6. The chance of my having a heart attack eventually can be strongly reduced by behavior that is under my control.
7. If I choose to exercise vigorously, I can diminish the frequency

of my irregular heart beats.

A woman who noticed small lumps along her groin worried about Hodgkin's disease, which had killed her grandmother. This was her list:

1. I have had these lumps for a long time without their changing size.
2. The doctor says that they are fibrotic lymph nodes and that she sees them all the time in healthy women.
3. Hodgkin's disease causes larger lymph nodes, often in clumps.
4. Hodgkin's disease is uniformly curable in the early stages.

It would be best if the health worrier were able to turn his or her attention elsewhere when the impulse to check erupts. With practice, this becomes possible. But as a substitute, checking a list of reassuring facts serves at least to leave the health worrier no worse than before. These are, after all, <u>reassuring</u> facts.

A written record of nightmare fantasies is also useful. Health worriers start off treatment not really believing they can ever worry less. It comes as a pleasant surprise to discover that thoughts that used to be too unpleasant to think about at all become dull and prosaic. The critical element in treatment is motivation. Any noticeable improvement will encourage the health worrier to persist in those unpleasant and sometimes prolonged exercises that lead ultimately to recovery.

Clinic meetings

Eight to ten patients meet with the group leader and three trained aides. Between meetings each patient meets with an assigned aide to facilitate cognitive-behavioral exercises and proper record keeping. The group — being a group — is affected by group dynamics. It is not uncommon for one or two patients to put off doing homework until motivated by group pressure, manifested in part by the encouragement and the visible improvement of some other members of the group. If the group is led by a psychologist, an internist or other medical specialist should be invited to attend at least one of the meetings to answer the medical questions that come up inevitably.

The meetings themselves tend to divide into two parts. A didactic portion is intended to correct as much as possible medical misconceptions, such as those discussed in <u>Worried Sick?</u>. The second part of each meeting addresses the particular fears of each patient and his or her progress. A detailed review of homework assignments is undertaken. Emphasis is placed on developing long term strategies to deal with those medical threats that have not yet surfaced but surely will in the future.

The first clinic meeting

Men and women often come to treatment with little understanding of why they worry too much. They tend to think of this problem as distinct from other emotional disorders. Sometimes they think that their worries are justified by the particular circumstances of their health. After filling out the health anxiety scale, they recognize that they must share some attitudes with other people, and even this much comes as a surprise; but they do not think of themselves as having a recognizable diagnostic problem.

Diagnosis in psychiatry is not worth a lot anyway. Conditions are defined on a descriptive basis, listing symptoms rather than causes; and there is considerable overlap. Still, it is comforting to know one has a familiar condition, along with many other people, and that that condition has a recognizable treatment and a potentially favorable outcome. The clinic program begins treatment, therefore, with a description of those emotional disorders which contribute to what we call health anxiety.

The following are excerpts from the Diagnostic and Statistical Manual of the American Psychiatric Association. They should be regarded as a consensus statement of what psychiatrists mean when they use these terms and should not be taken to refer to discrete clinical entities. (See the index of <u>Worried Sick?</u>)

Hypochondriasis

The critical relevant elements are the tendency to imagine the worst possible illness to explain current physical symptoms and, secondly, the inability to feel reassured by doctors.

Somatization Disorder

It is readily apparent that someone may have a great many physical symptoms without fulfilling exactly all the criteria to make this diagnosis. The essential element relevant to health anxiety is the tendency for some people to express emotional distress by developing physical symptoms such as headaches or stomach upset.

Panic Disorder

Panic disorder can occur by itself, but more commonly it leads to agoraphobia, which is a hesitancy to go into or remain in certain places.

Because panic attacks suggest to those that have them that they are about to faint, or have a heart attack or a seizure or some other physical calamity, they often lead to health anxiety.

Obsessive-Compulsive Disorder

The worries that occur to health worriers are usually obsessional in character. They are intrusive and persistent. Compulsive checking is an important aspect of the health worrier's behavior and the fear of germs or of contamination is often present in health anxiety.

Depression

The conventional wisdom is that all of the anxiety disorders listed here respond to some extent to anti-anxiety agents, particularly the serotonergic anti-depressants. But there is a much more significant and reliable response to these drugs when the cause of the anxiety is a concurrent depression. The presence of the so-called vegetative signs of depression are especially important. These are, first of all, a disorder of sleep marked by interrupted sleep and persistent early morning awakening. Upon awakening, the depressed person may or may not feel sad, but always feel bad in some way, often worried or physically agitated. This feeling wears off somewhat during the course of the day. Second, there is a disturbance of appetite, which can vary but is usually depressed to the point of losing weight. People so affected usually lose interest in sex at the same time.

It is important to delineate the symptoms of depression at the first meeting of the clinic because those patients who fulfill these criteria must be put on anti-depressant medications in order to participate effectively in a cognitive-behavioral treatment program. Because they are often afraid of these generally safe medications, special effort has to be made to encourage them.

Generalized Anxiety Disorder

Most health worriers will feel they fit into this category, along with some of the other categories. Some psychiatrists consider generalized anxiety disorder to be an illness or a group of illnesses very much as a major depression is. They use the same drugs to treat it. It may be more accurate, though, to think of people with this condition as having many discrete worries, so many as to occupy the affected person much of the day. It is usually more effective to deal with each worry one at a time rather than trying pharmacologically to lower the general level of anxiety. For similar reasons relaxation exercises are not quite to the point, although some treatment programs include them.

The great majority of patients who come to the health anxiety clinic have already been placed on anti-anxiety agents or anti-depressants without much improvement. However, many of them have had exaggerated reactions to these drugs and have stopped them prematurely or taken them in sub-clinical doses.

After dealing briefly with these various categories of emotional disorders, the clinic leader emphasizes the essential aspect of health anxiety, simply: the tendency to worry too much about one's health.

A number of clinical examples similar to those given in Worried Sick? are presented to give a sense of the variety of ways health worriers may come to medical attention. These accounts illustrate their tendency to go from doctor to doctor and worry about terrible diseases without much cause, and their tendency to engage in endless checking of their bodies. Usually patients in the current clinic readily identify with these others.

At this point the patients introduce themselves to each other. Typically patients are embarrassed initially by their concerns; and it is only when they receive a sympathetic hearing from the others, who often have the same worries, that they begin to feel comfortable. Over time, they develop a rooting interesting in each other's progress, which is very helpful.

Some explanation is offered of the causes of health anxiety:
1. Past experiences.
    A. Overprotective parents who communicate clearly their ideas about the precariousness of health.
    B. Exposure while growing up to a family member who had a serious, perhaps fatal, illness.
    C. Previous illnesses the patient may have had while growing up. These tend to have been prolonged and sometimes frightening to family members. Still, the great majority of children with asthma or juvenile diabetes grow up not worrying especially about their health; so something else is required.
2. Current or recent illnesses if they are unusually prolonged or

odd in some way. Patients seem more upset by obscure illness-es that are not readily understood by doctors than by the defi-nite diagnosis of a significant illness.

3. Doctors who make frightening remarks. It does not take much to scare people who are already for other reasons inclined to worry about their health; and some doctors say things that would scare anyone. Sometimes these warnings, or threats, are intended to get patients to follow through on some treatment recommendation. Other times a careless physician may muse aloud for no particular reason about some medical calamity the patient's symptoms call to mind, even though that possibility is far-fetched. There are some doctors who become truly fright-ened themselves because they know less than they should, and therefore order unnecessary tests or make draconian treatment recommendations.

4. Equivocal laboratory results. Someone who undergoes a great many laboratory tests will surely discover something sooner or later out of the normal range. These may be interpreted as a possible sign of illness and often set in motion additional testing or repeating the same test over and over again.

The factors mentioned above account for the underlying vul-nerability someone has to developing health anxiety, but they do not explain why it appears just when it does. The worry wheel is a diagram showing how this process begins and sustains itself.

The Worry Wheel
(See end of chapter – also see Worried Sick?)

In summary, some event, often inconsequential, starts the vul-nerable person thinking about the possibility of being sick. Self-examination leads to the discovery of equivocal signs of illness and provokes visits to the doctor. The doctor's response is never so unambiguous that the patient feels reassured. Tests are ordered which still further focus the patient's attention on the possibility of being ill. When these are reported back, the meaning of the results is often unclear and in any case provides no guarantee of being in good health. By now, the patient is worrying more rather than less. The process of worrying itself may provoke a wide variety of further symptoms such as pain from tensing muscles, or stomach cramps; and these are thought by the health worrier to reflect an underlying physical disorder. More worry occasions more checking and more visits to the doctor; and the whole process spirals out of control. Sometimes it comes to an end only long after the initial circumstance that started it has faded away. But the worry wheel is likely to start turning once again whenever a new trigger appears.

An explanation. of the principles of treatment.

In a way treatment is straightforward. The health worrier must confront his or her fears. Six ancillary principles of treatment are offered here in order to make this idea more concrete.

Six principles

1. Know the truth about yourself:
   - Your particular symptoms.
   - How you react to stress.
   - Know the truth about the illness you are likely to have and the illness you worry about
   - Knowing a little is scary.
   - Knowing a lot is reassuring. .
2. Confront your worst fears.
   - Thinking the unthinkable diminishes fear.
3. Avoid checking and the pursuit of empty reassurance. Learn how to distract yourself.
4. Think of the odds against being desperately ill, rather than the stakes. Consider the most likely illness rather than the worst.
5. Do not seek absolute certainty or safety.
6. Live in a healthy way.

Before the first meeting of the clinic is concluded, each patient is introduced to the aide he or she will be working with. They will meet together before the next clinic meeting. The purposes are as described previously:

1. To take a more detailed history.
2. To discover the most prominent nightmare fantasy.
3. To determine which particular disease or untoward medical events the patient fears.
4. To deter as far as possible any physical checking.
5. To enlist the support of family members.
6. To explain further the principles of treatment.

Problems that appear during the first week of the program:

The over-arching problem that appears in the first week of treatment and, to an extent, in subsequent weeks is cynicism. It is inevitable that a group of people who cannot trust their own physician will be doubtful of advice offered to them by another doctor, who is a stranger, especially when that advice is to go against their natural inclinations. The fact that this treatment for health anxiety is relatively new and not widely recognized is another reason to be skeptical. There is a logic, however, to these treatment recommendations; and patients will usually agree to the underlying principles, at least theoretically.

These are:

One should confront one's fears, systematically, rather than run from them. A child afraid of the monster under the bed will not overcome that fear once and for all, until he looks under the bed. Repeatedly. Even if the thought of looking under the bed— and, worse, the act of doing it— is really scary.

Secondly, it is always an advantage to know the truth. People can live more effectively if they truly understand themselves and their circumstances. Then they can plan properly. If health worriers are truly at risk, they should know about it, so they can protect themselves. If not, they should know that also, so they can stop worrying.

Reading about the feared disease, however disagreeable, can be justified in terms of these general principles. Harder to explain is the need to dwell on nightmare fantasies. This important bit of unpleasantness can only be understood in terms of a third principle: feelings fade. Everyone knows that grief, lust, the desire for revenge, and even fear, die out after a while if nothing new happens to sustain them; but most people, in the grip of a strong emotion, cannot believe that their particular passion or fear will ever fade. Health worriers have to expose themselves to their nightmare fantasies long enough to see for themselves that those thoughts lose their impact after an unexpectedly short time. But to know that, they have to be willing to try first.

The second clinic meeting

The second meeting and those subsequent follow the pattern of the first meeting. Part is given over to providing information. The more important part involves an examination of each patient's concerns and progress. Patients report their worries, their symptoms, and their practice sessions to each other and to the group. Each group has its own distinct character, but certain behaviors tend to recur. At one extreme is the enthusiast who goes immediately to the library to look up a feared disease and just as quickly takes up all the other difficult tasks required in treatment. Such a very unusual person gets better quickly. Somewhat more common, unfortunately, at the other extreme is the individual who comes to treatment sometimes at the urging of others with no expectation that it will work and who leaves as soon as it becomes obvious how much effort is required. The great majority of patients fall in between. Not trusting doctors in general, they do not start our program with any confidence. Also, they quickly discover that they are being asked to do things that are uncongenial and quite contrary to their natural inclinations. Often it takes weeks for a patient to stop checking his or her body, which seems easy enough to someone who does not have this problem. Similarly, patients put off contemplating their nightmare fantasies or reading about their feared disease. There is never time enough in someone's busy schedule to do something that is really unpleasant. Nevertheless, however tentative patients are at the beginning of treatment, obvious signs of progress begin to appear soon enough. And, as indicated before, most people get better.

The six principles of treatment mentioned before can be made still more explicit now. They translate into do's and don'ts.

<u>Do not</u>:

1. Do not examine your body except to the extent recommended by a doctor. Do not take your pulse, examine your stool or urine, check your temperature, look to see if your tongue is coated or if there are bags under yours eyes, or check to see if you are pale or flushed. Only examine your breasts or skin at those intervals prescribed by your doctor.
2. Do not ask your doctor or a family member the same question over and over again. Seek out new information as much as you can, but do not seek reassurance. Do not ask your spouse medical questions.
3. Do not encourage your doctor to order medical tests that he would not do on his own initiative. Do not ask for medication he would not otherwise think to prescribe.

<u>Do</u>:

1. Do research the disease, if any, your doctor thinks you have. Also, research the disease you are afraid you may have.
2. Do practice your various nightmare fantasies long enough for the emotional impact to disappear.
3. Do keep records of all the times you turned out not to be desperately ill.
4. Do exercise and eat properly (more of this later).

The remainder of the second meeting is given over largely to a discussion of how each person can follow these recommendations given their specific concerns. Some topics come up during all the meetings.

1. Where to go to find accurate medical information.
2. What to think about the latest medical threat reported in the newspaper.
3. How much of a risk is entailed by having family members with one particular disease or another.
4. How to practice in graduated steps confronting feared situations, such as hospital emergency rooms or having one's blood drawn.
5. How to keep the various records required by the treatment program.
6. How to manage difficulties in stopping the habit of checking.
7. The meaning of the latest laboratory tests.
8. The latest unsatisfactory encounter with a doctor or some other part of the medical establishment.
9. And, of course, the evolving saga of each patient's physical symptoms.
10. And each patient's current nightmare fantasy. The patients need to be reminded that they are supposed to contemplate these awful possibilities but also at each stage keep in mind the very small likelihood of these events coming to pass.

A typical problem of the second week of treatment.

Patients often persist stubbornly in the habit of checking, especially checking with their doctor. I mention in Worried Sick? health worriers who seek reassurance from their doctors and do not manage to leave their offices without feeling more worried; but there are many others who do feel relieved. Temporarily.

A young man reported that he had seen his physician 10 times in the previous year for different physical complaints, each of which vanished without a diagnosis being made and without treatment.

He said to me: "When I go to the doctor, and I'm worried, I do feel better when he tells me I'm okay. And when I ask my mom if she thinks I'm really sick, I know what she's going to say ahead of time; but I still feel better when she tells me I'm fine."

Checking provides a momentary relief of anxiety, otherwise no one would check. But asking a family member who is not knowledgable about medicine for empty reassurance is like getting a pat on the head. It has nothing to do with the search for the truth. It is demeaning to the person asking for reassurance and to the person giving it; and it serves to focus the health worrier's attention on his complaints. Asking a doctor the same question over and over is no better.

I pointed out to this young man that however comforted he may have been by visiting his doctor repeatedly for insignificant and transient symptoms, it did not lead to his feeling any more secure about his health. It was time to try something different.

The third clinic meeting

By now, some patients, perhaps most, will still be checking their body to some extent, although less. Some will have found reason to avoid considering their nightmare fantasies; but others will have thrown themselves into thinking and reading about these distressing possibilities so that their initial fears have faded. They have moved on to consider other fears that were under the surface. Some people are already feeling better and most are encouraging each other.

The didactic portion of the meeting is a discussion of how doctors diagnose illness (see pages 70 to 110 in Worried Sick?) and how to tell a good doctor from a bad doctor (see pages 78 to 86). The very few illnesses that require immediate emergency medical consultation, such as meningococcus meningitis or an acute coronary infarction, are discussed here.

Typical problems of the remaining weeks of the program.

Because the treatment of health anxiety is, at best, uncomfortable, patients often find one reason or another for not participating fully.

"I have family responsibilities and work responsibilities; and I can't find the hour a day you expect me to commit to working on this problem. Besides, my in-laws are visiting."

"It is simply too painful to read about cancer."

"I can't concentrate on anything until this laboratory test comes back," or "I'm worrying about a real illness right now."

"I don't think this is going to work. I don't think anything is going to work. I've had this problem all my life."

"No kidding, I'm too tired to exercise. I can barely make it up the steps to my bedroom."

I am sympathetic to these complaints. I recognize that whatever our problems may be, we continue to have other responsibilities which compete for our time. And I understand that we may get demoralized from time to time. Sometimes our fears are too great to accomplish what we would like to do all at once; but it should be possible to do a little. There is never an ideal time to read up on an unpleasant subject, or do homework. We have to do the best we can. Health anxiety is a stubborn condition. It may get better or worse, depending on the presence or absence of a physical illness; but it does not go away by itself.

The fourth clinic meeting

It is only at this point that all patients at last are spending considerable time looking up their most feared diseases and examining their nightmare fantasies. Some patients have given up checking only after being told to ask their physicians these explicit questions: "Is there any purpose served in my doing this checking?" "Am I endangering my health in any way by stopping this checking?" At this point, also, it may be possible to glimpse the underlying fears that lie beneath those initially apparent. They may include fears of physical deterioration or loneliness or helplessness — or a fear of severe pain or of one's children being orphaned. Some fears can be dispelled with more information. There are more complicated remedies for the fear of loneliness and helplessness. These lie in the subtle interplay of important personal relationships. They are an expression of personality and cannot be changed in the brief time of this clinic. But even a look into this labyrinth offers some insight into the meaning of life that each person must discover in order to be content.

The medical information presented in this meeting concerns medication (see pages 191 to 200 in <u>Worried Sick?</u>) and medical testing (see pages 110 to 120). As a rule health worriers are afraid of the side effects of drugs even though their safety has been tested at extraordinary expense by drug companies. Thus many prefer to take "natural" substances such as herbs. Many of these herbs are ineffectual or dangerous or both. Taking herbs is a bad idea. Here are some of the reasons:

1. The bottle that is labeled with the name of an herb may not contain any of that herb.
2. The amount of the herb said to be contained therein is not likely to be accurate, since it differs from manufacturer to manufacturer and batch to batch.
3. The chemical composition of most herbs is so complicated as to defy analysis. No one know whether or not the particular process undertaken to bring the drug to market inactivates whatever pharmacological effect the drug may have had.
4. Some herbs are, indeed, potent and dangerous. The ephedrine-like agents, can and do kill people. Other herbs have hormone-like effects and produce all those side effects that would come from taking hormones.
5. Some drugs have been shown to have been adulterated purposely with tranquilizers in order, presumably, to provide some noticeable effect.
6. Some of these agents, such as St. John's Wort, are particularly

dangerous when taken along with certain prescribed medicines.

7. The food and drug authority provides no oversight to the use of these drugs until after they have been shown to injure people. Injury may be caused to many different organs, especially the liver and kidney.

As in other areas of their lives, health worriers should be circumspect about using drugs but not afraid.

Whether or not to take any particular medicine should depend on a careful weighing of its effects and side effects. Placebo effects must be kept in mind. No general overall attitude towards drugs is justified.

Health worriers are troubled greatly by laboratory tests which may or may not have any significance. They look to tests and other investigative procedures to tell them definitely whether or not they have a certain disease. But few tests are truly definitive. If a test is ordered, they need to schedule it as quickly as possible and have it reported back as soon as possible. They need to understand that the test is not likely to tell them what they want to know. The test informs the doctor about what to do next.

The fifth clinic meeting

The group meeting at this point reflects a growing optimism. People have begun to feel better. What seemed initially an unpleasant and an unlikely treatment program seems now to offer some promise. Even so, most patients find some reason some of the time not to practice. Most patients are distracted still to some extent at least by their particular symptoms. Therefore, something of a lecture is presented at this point by a physician who describes in general terms how to distinguish gastroesophageal pain and chest wall pain from a heart attack, ordinary headache from a brain tumor, fibrocystic breast disease from cancer, leukemia from simple bruising or swollen lymph glands, the light headedness of an anxiety attack from true vertigo, and so on.

Health worriers who confuse these conditions <u>even after reading about them</u> can be seen to make certain characteristic errors:

1. They focus on the nonspecific symptoms, such as fatigue, that they experience and share with the serious illness and gloss over those defining symptoms of the serious illness that they do not have.

2. They do not realize that if the particular symptoms they have were to be caused by the disease they dread, many other symptoms that they do not have would have occurred first.

3. They think when they have a little of a symptom, such as enlarged lymph nodes, they are half-way along to developing a serious symptom, such as greatly enlarged lymph nodes. The former are produced by many inconsequential diseases. They are a symptom of no importance.

4. They become afraid if they fall into some category of increased risk of a disease even if the risk is still tiny. If there is an illness in the family that doubles their risk of getting it from one in a thousand to one in five hundred, this fact should not bother them. Similarly, there are many circumstances of environment that raise the risk of an illness from teeny to tiny and are not worth worrying about, whatever they have read to the contrary.

5. They make judgments on medical matters, particularly on the likelihood of untoward medical events, based on personal experience. Personal experience includes what happened, or what they think happened, to friends or to friends of their friends. Like any other gossip, these accounts tend to be dramatic and exaggerated.

If is odd that many patients who are so afraid of becoming sick and possibly dying should not take those measures which are known to lessen the risks of cancer and heart disease and many of the debilitating diseases of middle and old age. Since the exaggerated worry that characterizes health anxiety is partly a response to a sense of helplessness in the face of danger, it is important in a program of treatment to outline what can be done to prevent serious illness and premature death.

1. Smoking cigarettes is the single most unhealthy thing anyone can do. Not only is smoking responsible for at least one third of all cardiovascular and cancer deaths, it leads to miserable diseases such as emphysema that can ruin life. Stopping smoking even after many years, can lower much of this risk.

2. Nutritional factors have a very considerable effect on health. The Mediterranean diet has been shown to diminish the risk from heart disease and premature death from other causes too. The diet emphasizes vegetables, fish, olive oil and moderate amounts of wine. The benefits of the diet probably do not derive from an effect on blood cholesterol. Whether or not to take additional vitamins is still controversial. The Food and Drug Administration empannels a group of experts every so often to make recommendations in this regard; and, with a few exceptions, they have chosen not to recommend taking vitamins over and above what is present in a normal diet. But they are motivated to a considerable extent by the fear of giving advice which turns out later to be wrong. For example, many nutritionists used to recommend taking beta carotene supplements, an antioxidant. Further research suggested that beta carotene may compete in the body with other more important carotenoids present in food. It may actually raise the risk of cancer rather than lower it. Similarly, it seems that the long emphasis on lowering the level of fat in the diet leads neither to a lower rate of obesity or to a lower over – all death rate. Because these authorities find it embarrassing to change their minds publicly, they hesitate much longer than they should to make recommendations and even longer before they change them. They finally decided to add folic acid, a B vitamin, to

bread only years after it had been shown to lower the risk to pregnant women of giving birth to babies with neural tube defects. But the rest of us have to live in the present guided by the best information we have now, even if the future should prove us to be wrong.

Most people probably do not eat a proper diet; and certainly older people have been shown to be vitamin deficient. Except in unusual circumstances, these substances are harmless in amounts greater than those generally recommended currently. There is reason to think that the risk of many serious illnesses would be lowered by taking a multivitamin without iron. Within limits, extra vitamin C and vitamin E may be helpful; and there are probably benefits in taking still other B vitamins such as folic acid and B 12. Small amounts of selenium have been shown to lower the risk of prostate cancer; and calcium lowers the risk of osteoporosis, hypertension and probably colon cancer. Of these substances only calcium, which may cause constipation, has any discernible side effect. The evidence for and against taking extra vitamins and minerals has filled a library. It is reasonable for someone who is inclined to take them to check first with his or her physician.

3. It is unhealthy and demoralizing to be obese, and not only because of social prejudices against fat people. The bad effects of obesity on arthritis and heart disease, among other diseases, are well known. It is probably healthier to be in the lower part of the normal weight range. It is known that caloric restriction can extend life in animals not otherwise nutritionally deficient.

4. There is a small but growing number of medicines that can be taken by normal people to lower the risk of developing certain diseases like osteoporosis or coronary artery disease. People should not shy away from these drugs as a matter of principle.

5. Many of our patients are at an age where the commonest cause of death are accidents and violence. If they use seat belts systematically, their risk of a serious injury from an auto-

mobile accident will be cut down considerably. Having a gun in the house for "protection" has been shown to increase greatly the chance of dying violently. Guns should be removed form the home. Also, health worriers should be willing to consider the possibility that they may be depressed. It is a common and treatable disorder; and it may lead to suicide. There are more than 30,000 deaths in this country every year from suicide.

6. Exercise. Physical inactivity is an independent risk factor for heart disease and for other medical problems. Exercise also has an effect on morale. Someone doing well in a competitive sport is less likely to regard himself or herself as physically impaired. In addition, someone experiencing shortness of breath, an accelerated heart rate, dry mouth and unsteadiness as the result of vigorous exercise is less likely to attribute these symptoms at other times to the presence of some hidden medical problem.

The sixth clinic meeting

The last clinic meeting is usually delayed by a week to see if new medical problems have surfaced and if patients have continued the exercises and record keeping encouraged in the program. It is a chance to judge progress and make plans for the future. The principal purpose of this meeting is to summarize those strategies that can be used to deal with the next medical worry.

The next time patients are confronted with a medical threat they are likely still to have the same first reaction, becoming more upset than is justified by the nature of that threat. Attitudes that have developed over the course of a lifetime tend to reassert themselves. Of course, there may be fewer occasions to feel threatened in the first place. They may know too much about a particular illness to worry about it anymore, even in the face of the sort of symptoms or news report that might previously have upset them. But given a new medical problem, they may very well think first once again of the worst possible condition and feel that same sinking feeling. But then a new process should start in motion. They ask, is this awful condition really likely? Are there other possible explanations for this symptom? Where can I go to get more information about this problem? Is this symptom any different really from what I experienced the last time I went to a doctor? Can I safely wait a while before I call or visit the doctor? Is this the kind of condition that may go away on its own? They turn to the records they have kept in the past. Is this new symptom really new? Is this likely to be a false alarm as it turned out to be the last 40 or 50 times?

After calming down somewhat, as they will, health worriers, or former health worriers, find it possible now to distract themselves with other thoughts and activities. They still have to fight the urge to ask their spouses for a medical opinion; but if they do, it is likely to be only once and not over and over. Since they are out of the habit of worrying they will find themselves forgetting just what was upsetting to them only a few minutes or a few hours before. On those occasions when the threat is real enough to continue to preoccupy them, they know to read about the condition promptly, usually with the result that they find reason to feel secure. If not, they can once again sit down to consider the "what if. . .well, then..." possibilities that make up a nightmare fantasy.

It is hard to know when health anxiety is cured since it shows up only from time to time anyway, and because sometimes severe medical problems can develop that would frighten anyone. But it is readily apparent that patients who have gone through the program worry less in general, and when a threat does loom up suddenly, they confront it promptly. If some medical intervention or treatment needs to be done, they do it quickly and no longer dwell on what might have been or what could be in the future.

Results of Treatment

Health anxiety waxes and wanes depending to some extent on circumstances. It is difficult, therefore, to determine the effectiveness of treatment over a long period of time. It is also difficult to arrange a scientific test of a psychological treatment, since that would require a control group and a complicated test protocol. Besides, it is possible that some patients report themselves as improved simply to please the treating therapist. Others, for their own reasons, may not acknowledge to their families, and to the world in general, just how much they have improved. Nevertheless, the following report of the first 100 patients to attend the health anxiety clinic at White Plains Hospital might be regarded as an appropriate guide to treatment success. At the conclusion of the clinic:

> 7 said they were improved completely
> 25 said they were improved very much
> 43 said they were improved moderately and
> 25 said they were improved a little.

From the perspective of a few years later, there are at least a few, I can attest to personally, who are completely well.

THE ANXIETY & PHOBIA TREATMENT CENTER
HEALTH ANXIETY PROGRAM

FORM A

How many times a day does a health worry occur to you? _____

Do your health worries interfere with your life?

They spoil much of my life _____

They interfere a great deal _____

They interfere to a moderate degree _____

They interfere somewhat _____

They interfere not at all _____

Name_____ Date _____

The Anxiety & Phobia Center
White Plains Hospital Center

FORM B

Chief Complaint _____

Tentative Diagnosis _____

HEALTH ANXIETY SCALE

	Yes	No
Do you feel that you are likely to get sick more frequently than others, or are likely to get sicker than others when you do get sick?		
Do you think a lot about the possibility of getting illnesses that run in your family?		
When you develop physical symptoms, do you immediately contemplate the most serious illness that could explain these symptoms?		
Do you often think how terrible it would be for you or your children if you were to die prematurely?		
Are you under the impression that it is very important to get to a doctor at the first sign of getting sick?		
Do you visit doctors much more frequently than you really need to in order to be reassured about your health?		
Do you avoid doctors because you are frightened about what they might discover?		
Do you leave the doctor's office sometimes unsure of what he said or meant because you were nervous when he spoke to you?		
Although you know medical opinions can never be certain, do you nevertheless ask you doctor questions such as "are you sure I don't have cancer ... or AIDS ... or high blood pressure, etc.?" Is it hard for the doctor to reassure you?		
Do you ask what the cause of a symptom is even when the doctor has told you that that symptom is inconsequential?		

38

Do you ask your doctor to do medical tests in order "to be sure" even if the doctor is not otherwise inclined to order such tests?		
Do you worry for days ahead of time about routine tests such as a mammogram?		
Do you worry when a laboratory test result falls outside the normal range?		
Do you hesitate to take prescribed medicines because of concern about side effects?		
Are you more sensitive to medication than other people?		
Are you more inclined to take "natural" substances, such as herbs, rather than prescribed medicines?		
Do you worry when you have trouble sleeping or if your bowels are irregular?		
Do you check parts of your body over and over again looking for an abnormality such as a lump?		
Do you often suffer palpitations?		
Do you ask other people, such as a spouse, whether you are looking a little better today or a little worse?		
Do you worry about germs or about catching someone else's illness?		
Do you worry about very unlikely diseases such as a brain aneurysm that tend to lurk silently and may suddenly kill you?		
Are you preoccupied much of the time with thoughts of becoming ill or dying to the point, sometimes, where family members feel obligated to reassure you?		
Do you feel your health worries are foolish?		

THE WORRY WHEEL

1. A predilection to be fearful

2. A trigger (perceived threat) – perhaps an illness or even a friend's illness, perhaps only watching a television program.

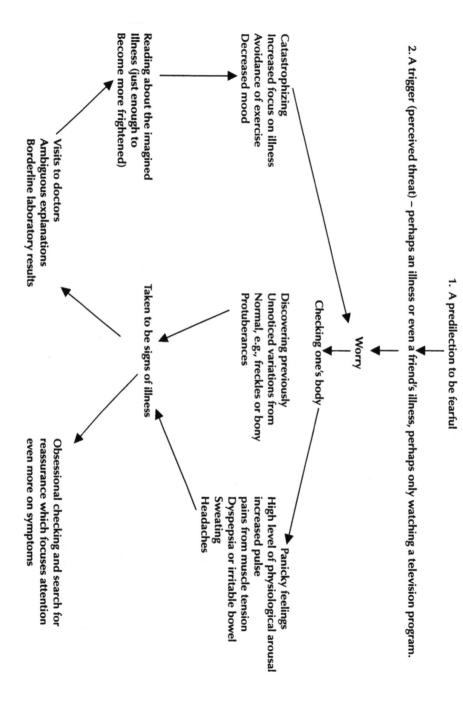

Worry

Checking one's body

Panicky feelings
High level of physiological arousal
increased pulse
pains from muscle tension
Dyspepsia or irritable bowel
Sweating
Headaches

Discovering previously
Unnoticed variations from
Normal, e.g., freckles or bony
Protuberances

Taken to be signs of illness

Obsessional checking and search for
reassurance which focuses attention
even more on symptoms

Catastrophizing
Increased focus on illness
Avoidance of exercise
Decreased mood

Reading about the imagined
illness (just enough to
Become more frightened)

Visits to doctors
Ambiguous explanations
Borderline laboratory results

40

The symptom I have:	The worry I have in Connection with this symptom:	What happened to this symptom:

The symptom I have:	The worry I have in Connection with this symptom:	What happened to this symptom:

The symptom I have:	The worry I have in Connection with this symptom:	What happened to this symptom:

The symptom I have:	The worry I have in Connection with this symptom:	What happened to this symptom:

The symptom I have:	The worry I have in Connection with this symptom:	What happened to this symptom:

The symptom I have:	The worry I have in Connection with this symptom:	What happened to this symptom:

The symptom I have:	The worry I have in Connection with this symptom:	What happened to this symptom:

The symptom I have:	The worry I have in Connection with this symptom:	What happened to this symptom:

The symptom I have:	The worry I have in Connection with this symptom:	What happened to this symptom:

The symptom I have:	The worry I have in Connection with this symptom:	What happened to this symptom:

The symptom I have:	The worry I have in Connection with this symptom:	What happened to this symptom:

The symptom I have:	The worry I have in Connection with this symptom:	What happened to this symptom:

The symptom I have:	The worry I have in Connection with this symptom:	What happened to this symptom:

The symptom I have:	The worry I have in Connection with this symptom:	What happened to this symptom:

The symptom I have:	The worry I have in Connection with this symptom:	What happened to this symptom:

The symptom I have:	The worry I have in Connection with this symptom:	What happened to this symptom:

The symptom I have:	The worry I have in Connection with this symptom:	What happened to this symptom:

The symptom I have:	The worry I have in Connection with this symptom:	What happened to this symptom:

The symptom I have:	The worry I have in Connection with this symptom:	What happened to this symptom:

The symptom I have:	The worry I have in Connection with this symptom:	What happened to this symptom:

The symptom I have:	The worry I have in Connection with this symptom:	What happened to this symptom:

The symptom I have:	The worry I have in Connection with this symptom:	What happened to this symptom:

The symptom I have:	The worry I have in Connection with this symptom:	What happened to this symptom:

The symptom I have:	The worry I have in Connection with this symptom:	What happened to this symptom:

The symptom I have:	The worry I have in Connection with this symptom:	What happened to this symptom:

The symptom I have:	The worry I have in Connection with this symptom:	What happened to this symptom:

The symptom I have:	The worry I have in Connection with this symptom:	What happened to this symptom:

The symptom I have:	The worry I have in Connection with this symptom:	What happened to this symptom:

The symptom I have:	The worry I have in Connection with this symptom:	What happened to this symptom:

The symptom I have:	The worry I have in Connection with this symptom:	What happened to this symptom:

Lightning Source UK Ltd.
Milton Keynes UK
UKHW030606281118
333086UK00005B/156/P

9 780981 484358